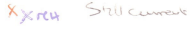

# New and expectant mothers at work

## A guide for employers

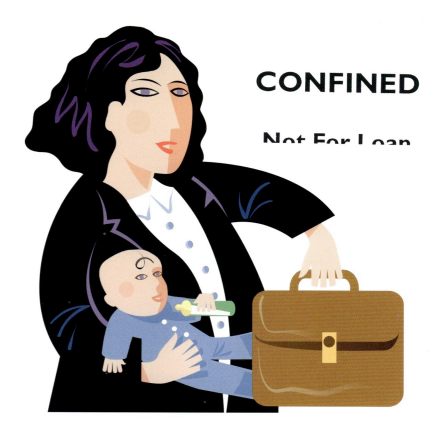

CONFINED

Not For Loan

HSE BOOKS

**New and expectant mothers at work**
A guide for employers

© *Crown copyright 2002*
*First published 1994*
*Second edition 2002*

**ISBN 0 7176 2583 4**

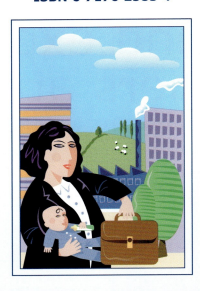

This guidance is issued by the Health and Safety Executive. Following the guidance is not compulsory and you are free to take other action. But if you do follow the guidance you will normally be doing enough to comply with the law. Health and safety inspectors seek to secure compliance with the law and may refer to this guidance as illustrating good practice.

# Contents

**New and expectant mothers at work**
A guide for employers

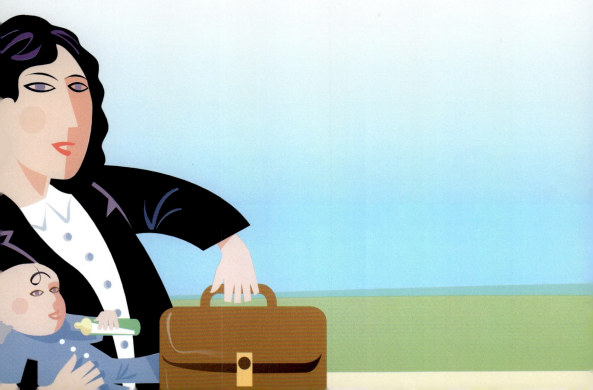

# Introduction

1 Pregnancy should not be regarded as ill health. It is part of everyday life and its health and safety implications can be adequately addressed by normal health and safety management procedures.

2 Many women work while they are pregnant and may return to work while they are still breastfeeding. Some hazards in the workplace may affect the health and safety of new and expectant mothers and of their child(ren). Therefore, working conditions normally considered acceptable may no longer be so during pregnancy and while breastfeeding.

3 In most cases pregnancy usually goes undetected for the first 4-6 weeks. It is important for employers to identify hazards and risks for all female employees of childbearing age. They should also take into account that some hazards can present more of a risk at different stages of the pregnancy.

4 The law at present requires employers to assess risks to their employees, including new and expectant mothers, and to do what is reasonably practicable to control those risks. Exposure limits for hazardous substances and other agents are set at levels which should not put a pregnant or breastfeeding worker, or her child, at risk. (In some cases, there are lower exposure levels for pregnant workers, or for women of childbearing capacity, than for other workers.) Controlling common workplace risks appropriately will reduce the need for special action for new and expectant mothers.

5 This guidance takes you through the actions you will need to take, provides information on known risks to new and expectant mothers, and gives advice on what you need to do to comply with the law (Appendix 1). There is also some advice on other aspects of pregnancy which may affect work (Appendix 2). Although these are not covered by legal requirements, we recommend you take them into account.

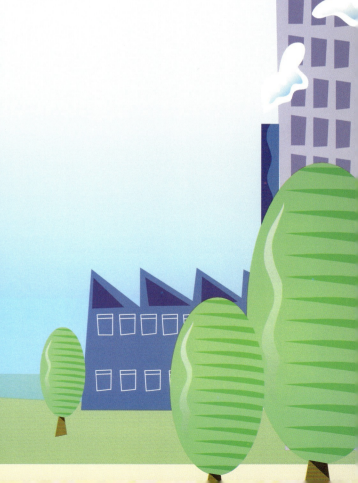

2

**New and expectant mothers at work**
A guide for employers

# Legal requirements

6 The health and safety of new and expectant mothers at work is covered by the Management of Health and Safety at Work Regulations 1999 (MHSW).[1] You are required to assess risks to all your employees and to do what is reasonably practicable to control those risks. You are also required to take into account risks to new and expectant mothers when assessing risks in your work activity.

7 If you cannot avoid a risk by other means, you are specifically required to make changes to the working conditions or hours of a new or expectant mother, offer her suitable alternative work, or if that is not possible suspend her for as long as necessary to protect her health and safety and that of her baby.

8 Where an employee works nights and produces a certificate from a registered medical practitioner or a registered midwife showing that it is necessary for her health and safety not to work nights, you should suspend her from that work for the period identified in the certificate. The Employment Rights Act 1996[41] requires that suitable alternative daytime work on the same terms and conditions should be offered before suspending the woman from work (further information on this Act and the Sex Discrimination Act 1975[43] is provided in Appendix 3).

9 You only have to follow the requirements outlined in paragraphs 7-8 once you have been notified in writing that a worker is pregnant, has given birth in the previous six months, or is breastfeeding. You may request, in writing, a certificate from a registered medical practitioner or a registered midwife confirming the pregnancy. If, within a reasonable period of time, the employee has not produced the certificate you are not required to continue following the requirements.

10 Under the Workplace (Health, Safety and Welfare) Regulations 1992[2] you are required to provide suitable facilities for workers who are pregnant or breastfeeding to rest.

## Definitions

11 The phrase 'new or expectant mother' means an employee who is pregnant, who has given birth within the previous six months, or who is breastfeeding.

12 'Given birth' is defined in the Management of Health and Safety at Work Regulations as 'delivered a living child or, after 24 weeks of pregnancy, a stillborn child'.

## What you need to do

13 In assessing risks to your employees you need to specifically consider workers who are new or expectant mothers, and to take action to ensure that they are not exposed to any significant risk. You will also need to ensure that the person carrying out the assessment is competent and able to take due account of all relevant information.

14 The flowchart at Figure 1 shows what you must do if you have female workers of childbearing age.

# Stage one – Initial risk assessment

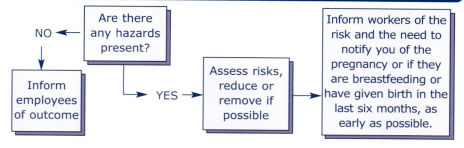

NO ← Are there any hazards present?

Inform employees of outcome

YES → Assess risks, reduce or remove if possible →

Inform workers of the risk and the need to notify you of the pregnancy or if they are breastfeeding or have given birth in the last six months, as early as possible.

# Stage two – On notification of pregnancy, birth or breastfeeding

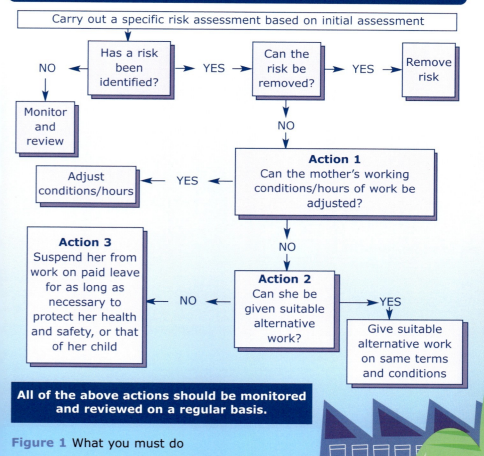

Carry out a specific risk assessment based on initial assessment

NO ← Has a risk been identified? → YES → Can the risk be removed? → YES → Remove risk

Monitor and review

NO ↓

**Action 1**
Can the mother's working conditions/hours of work be adjusted?

Adjust conditions/hours ← YES ←

NO ↓

**Action 3**
Suspend her from work on paid leave for as long as necessary to protect her health and safety, or that of her child

← NO ←

**Action 2**
Can she be given suitable alternative work? → YES ↓

Give suitable alternative work on same terms and conditions

**All of the above actions should be monitored and reviewed on a regular basis.**

**Figure 1** What you must do

# Stage one – Initial risk assessment

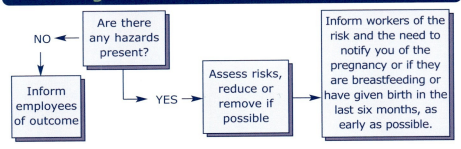

**Figure 2** Initial risk assessment

## *Stage one*

15 When you do the initial risk assessment (see Figure 2), you must take into account any hazards and risks to females of childbearing age. This includes new and expectant mothers. Risks include those to the unborn child or the child of a woman who is still breastfeeding and not just risks to the mother herself. You can get more information about risk assessment in HSE's *Five steps to risk assessment* leaflet.[3]

### i) Look for hazards

16 The physical, biological and chemical agents, processes and working conditions which may affect the health and safety of new or expectant mothers are set out in Appendix 1. They include the following possible hazards.

**Physical risks**

- Movements and postures
- Manual handling
- Shocks and vibrations
- Noise
- Radiation (ionising and non-ionising)
- Compressed air and diving
- Underground mining work

**Biological agents**

- Infectious diseases

**Chemical agents, including:**

- Toxic chemicals
- Mercury
- Antimitotic (cytotoxic) drugs
- Pesticides
- Carbon monoxide
- Lead

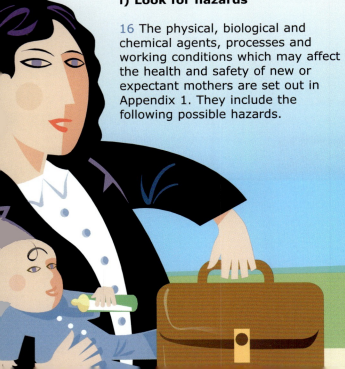

## Working conditions

- Facilities (including rest rooms)
- Mental and physical fatigue and working hours
- Stress (including postnatal depression)
- Passive smoking
- Temperature
- Working with visual display units (VDUs)
- Working alone
- Work at heights
- Travelling
- Violence
- Working and personal protective equipment
- Nutrition

All of these are listed in the annexes to the European Directive on the health and safety of pregnant workers (92/85/EEC)[4] and the European Commission's guidelines.[5]

17 Many of these are already covered by specific health and safety regulations, eg Control of Lead at Work (CLAW),[6] Control of Substances Hazardous to Health Regulations (COSHH).[7] The table in Appendix 1 includes details of the specific regulations and other guidance available (where they apply).

18 If any of these hazards are present in your workplace you should refer to the relevant regulations or guidance for information on what you should do. See *References*.

## ii) Decide who might be harmed and how

19 Your risk assessment may show that there is a substance or work process in your workplace that could damage the health or safety of new and expectant mothers or their children. You will need to bear in mind that there could be different risks depending on whether workers are pregnant, have recently given birth, or are breastfeeding. You should also take account of the needs of employees with atypical work patterns (eg shift workers), and those who may not be your employees but are working under your direction or control (eg contractors).

20 You should take into account that there is usually a period of between 4-6 weeks during which a worker may not be aware that she is pregnant and is therefore unable or reluctant to inform her employer. You can overcome this problem by taking special care in respect of all workers by reducing their exposure to harmful agents.

## iii) Consult your employees and inform them of any risk

21 You must consult your employees on any health and safety matters, including decisions you are planning to make which might affect their health and safety. You should inform your employees or their representatives of what is being proposed, allowing them time to express their views and should take account of their views before you reach a final decision.

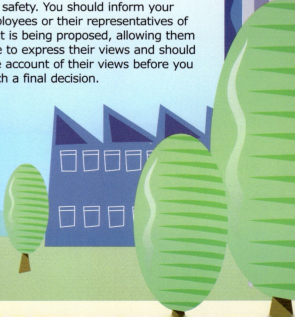

22 If your assessment does reveal a risk you should tell all female employees of childbearing age about the potential risks if they are, or could in the future be, pregnant or breastfeeding. You should also explain what you plan to do to make sure that new and expectant mothers are not exposed to the risks that could cause them harm. It is important that you reiterate the need for written notification of pregnancy, or that they are breastfeeding or have given birth in last six months, as early as possible.

23 Figure 3 shows an example of a completed risk assessment in a small office.

## *Stage two*

24 When an employee notifies you that she is pregnant, you should carry out a specific risk assessment based on the outcome of your initial risk assessment and any medical advice received on the health of the employee. As with the initial risk assessment, this should be conducted by a 'competent person' who is able to take account of all the relevant information. See Figure 4.

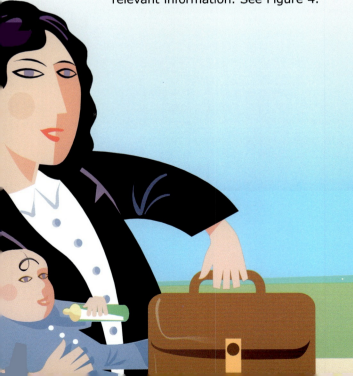

# Assessment of possible risks to new and expectant mothers

This note summarises the initial risk assessment that has been carried out concerning the risks to new and expectant mothers in our office.

We do not equate pregnancy with ill health. The intention is simply to prevent risks to the expectant or new mother and to the child from work which would not usually produce such risk. A number of factors have been considered, as set out below, and will be regularly reviewed or sooner if the need becomes apparent.

## Rest facilities

The first-aid room may be used for rest purposes. In view of its remote location you should tell another member of staff if you are using it.

## Seating

A chair which is suitably adjustable is an important part of achieving correct posture when working at a desk and in particular at a computer workstation. A DSE (Display Screen Equipment) assessment, which included posture, was carried out for all staff in the office. You should request a further assessment or review if you experience discomfort or cannot achieve correct posture.

## Hazards identified

*Manual handling*
Pregnant and postnatal mothers are at much greater risk than usual from manual handling. They should not lift heavy loads, such as single packs of paper or parcels. If heavy items such as post bags, typewriters or furniture need to be moved a risk assessment will be needed. Expectant and new mothers should not normally be involved in such tasks.

Tasks that could usually be done safely, without difficulty, may become inadvisable. It is recommended that you should avoid tasks which involve stretching up, down or out, for example retrieving items from under desks or from between cabinets, particularly when it is uncomfortable to do so.

*Continuous sitting*
Tea breaks and lunch breaks are available to all employees.

**Carried out by**: Mr J Bloggs

**Date**: 10.05.2002

**Review date set for**: 10.08.2002

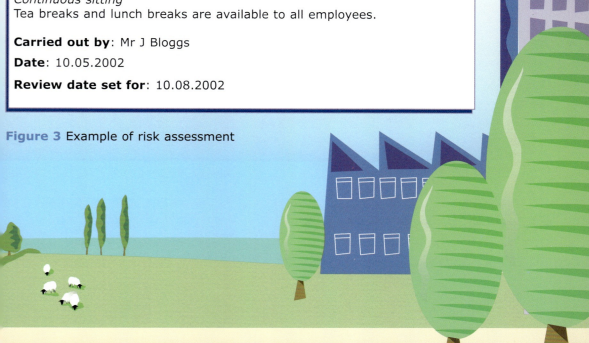

**Figure 3** Example of risk assessment

## Stage two – On notification of pregnancy, birth or breastfeeding

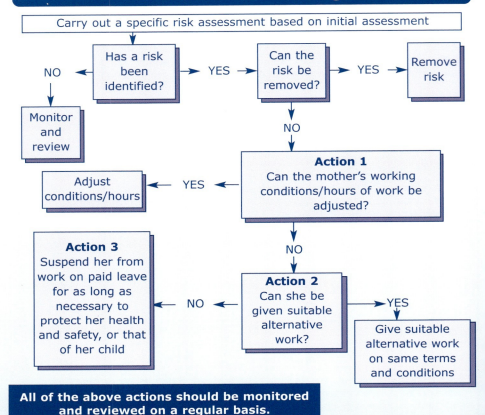

Carry out a specific risk assessment based on initial assessment

Has a risk been identified?

NO → Monitor and review

YES → Can the risk be removed?

YES → Remove risk

NO →

**Action 1** Can the mother's working conditions/hours of work be adjusted?

YES → Adjust conditions/hours

NO →

**Action 2** Can she be given suitable alternative work?

YES → Give suitable alternative work on same terms and conditions

NO → **Action 3** Suspend her from work on paid leave for as long as necessary to protect her health and safety, or that of her child

**All of the above actions should be monitored and reviewed on a regular basis.**

**Figure 4** On notification of pregnancy, birth or breastfeeding

25 If there is a significant risk at work to the health and safety of a new or expectant mother, which goes beyond the level of risk found outside the workplace, then you must take the following actions to remove her from the risk:

**Action 1** temporarily adjust her working conditions and/or hours of work; or if it is not reasonable to do so, or would not avoid the risk:

**Action 2** offer her suitable alternative work (at the same rate of pay) if available; or if that is not feasible, you must:

**Action 3** suspend her from work on paid leave for as long as necessary to protect her health and safety, and that of her child.

26 These actions are only necessary where, as the result of a risk assessment, there is genuine concern. If there is any doubt, you may want to seek professional advice on what the risks are, and whether they arise from work, before offering alternative employment or paid leave. Any alternative work you offer should also be subject to a risk assessment.

### iv) Keep risks under review

27 You will need to keep your risk assessments for new and expectant mothers under review. Although hazards are likely to remain constant, the risk of damage to the unborn child as a result of a hazard will vary at different stages of a pregnancy. Dexterity, agility, co-ordination, speed of movement, and reach may be impaired because of increasing size.

# Breastfeeding

28 There are other risks to consider for workers who are breastfeeding. For example, organic mercury can be transferred from blood to milk causing a potential risk to the newborn baby if the mother is highly exposed before and during pregnancy. These risks are listed in Appendix 1.

29 You will need to ensure, on receiving written notification that a worker is breastfeeding, that she is not exposed to risks that could damage her health and safety and that of her child for as long as she continues to breastfeed. The regulations do not put a time limit on breastfeeding. It is for women themselves to decide how long they

wish to breastfeed, depending on individual circumstances. The Department of Health recommends breastfeeding for the first four to six months. After that time, breastfeeding can be continued along with the safe introduction of solid food.

30 It is good practice to provide a healthy and safe environment for nursing mothers to express and store milk. These facilities could be included in the suitable resting facilities you must provide for pregnant and breastfeeding mothers (see *Legal requirements*).

31 Where workers continue to breastfeed for many months after birth, you will want to review the risks regularly. Where you identify risks, you will need to continue to follow the actions outlined above and in the flowchart (see Figure 1) in order to avoid exposure to risk for as long as it threatens the health and safety of the breastfeeding worker and her child.

32 Where employers are controlling risks in line with the regulations, it is unlikely that workers who continue breastfeeding will be exposed to risks which give rise to the need for them to be offered alternative work or given paid leave. If you have any doubts, you may wish to call on professional advice from an occupational health specialist.

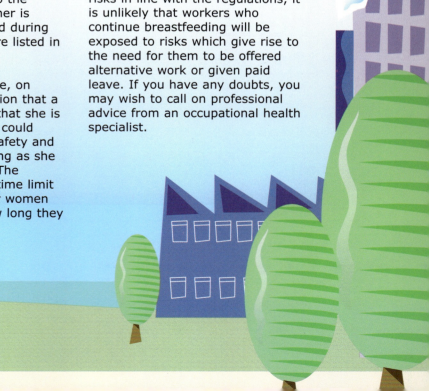

# Night work

33 You need to give special consideration to new and expectant mothers who work at night. Regulations require that if an employee who is a new or expectant mother works at night, and has a medical certificate stating that night work could affect her health and safety, you must either:

a) offer her suitable alternative daytime work, if any is available; or if that is not reasonable

b) suspend her from work, on paid leave, for as long as is necessary to protect her health and safety and that of her child.

34 You are only required to do this if the risk arises from work. HSE experts are not aware of any additional risks to pregnant or breastfeeding workers or their child(ren) from working at night per se.

# Maternity rights

35 Maternity rights fall into four main categories:

- time off work for antenatal care;
- maternity leave;
- maternity pay; and

- protection against unfair treatment or dismissal.

36 There are two maternity benefits available to pregnant working women:

- Statutory Maternity Pay - paid by employers; and
- Maternity Allowance - paid by the Department for Work and Pensions.

37 You can find more information in the Department of Trade and Industry's leaflet *Maternity rights - a guide for employers and employees;*[8] on their 'Tailored interactive guidance on employment rights' website www.tiger.gov.uk; on the Inland Revenue website www.ir.gov.uk; and for maternity allowance the Department for Work and Pensions' website www.dwp.gov.uk.

# Confidentiality

38 Medical advice, reports and certificates should take working conditions into consideration. The confidentiality concerning a woman's pregnancy means an employer should not make it known that she is pregnant if she does not wish it to be known or if she does not consent to it. Exceptionally, in certain circumstances, it may be necessary to take steps (including limited disclosure) to protect her health and safety, but this should be done with the woman's agreement following consultation.

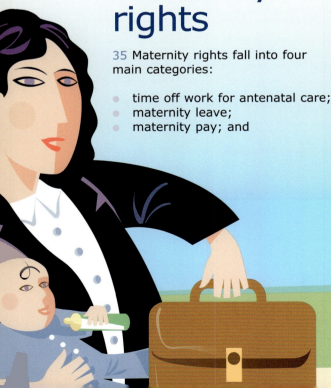

# Case studies

39  These case studies provide examples of good and bad practice when an employer has been notified of a pregnancy.

## Good practice

A care worker notified her employer of her pregnancy. The employer looked back at the outcome of the initial risk assessment, which had identified that a possible risk for pregnant women was exposure to acts of violence (eg difficult patients). The employer then conducted a specific risk assessment for the pregnant worker, who dealt with patients who were difficult and on occasion violent. As a result the employer offered the care worker suitable alternative work at the same salary and reviewed the assessment at regular intervals. The employee accepted the alternative work and had a risk free pregnancy. Following her maternity leave the employee returned to work.

## Good practice

An office worker notified her employer of her pregnancy. The employer hired an occupational health professional consultant to conduct a specific risk assessment. The consultant identified that there were problems with the pregnant worker's hours and workload, as well as certain physical aspects of her workstation. The employer adjusted the workstation as advised and reduced the employee's workload so that she was able to continue to work the same hours at the same rate of pay. The employer monitored and reviewed the assessment at regular intervals throughout the employee's pregnancy. The employee had a risk free pregnancy and returned to work at end of her maternity leave.

## Bad practice

On notifying her employer of pregnancy, a sales worker was given extra work and put under pressure to exceed her sales targets prior to going on maternity leave. The pregnant worker suffered a miscarriage and was signed off from work due to stress.

The employer was taken to an Employment Tribunal where the judgement found that they were in breach of health and safety legislation for not conducting a specific risk assessment. They were also found to be in breach of the Sex Discrimination Act and the Employment Rights Acts.

Much time and expense could have been saved if the employer had conducted a risk assessment (see paragraphs 15-27).

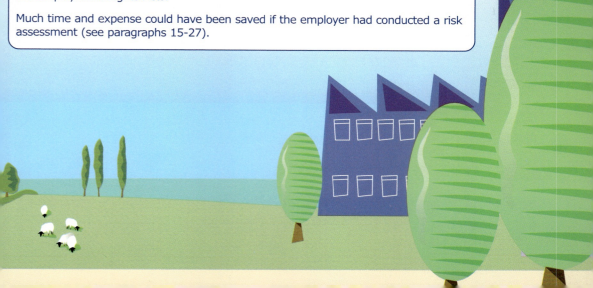

# Appendix 1 - Hazards, risk

This includes physical, chemical and biological agents and working conditions listed in Annex

| List of agents/working conditions | What is the risk? |
|---|---|

**PHYSICAL RISKS** - where these are regarded as agents causing foe*

| | |
|---|---|
| **Movements and postures** | The nature and extent of any risks of injury or ill health resulting from movements or posture during and after pregnancy will depend on a number of factors, including:<br>• the nature, duration and frequency of tasks/movements;<br>• the pace, intensity and variety of work;<br>• patterns of working time and rest breaks;<br>• ergonomic factors and the general working environment; and<br>• the suitability and adaptability of any work equipment involved.<br><br>Hormonal changes in women who are pregnant or have recently given birth can affect the ligaments, increasing susceptibility to injury. The resulting injury may not be apparent until some time after the birth.  You should also pay particular attention to women who may handle loads during the three months following a return to work after childbirth.<br><br>Postural problems can arise at different stages of pregnancy, and on returning to work, depending on the individual and her working conditions.  These problems may increase as the pregnancy progresses, especially if the work involves awkward movements or long periods of standing or sitting in one position.<br><br>**Standing**: Continuous standing during the working day may lead to dizziness, faintness, and fatigue.  It can also contribute to an increased risk of premature childbirth and miscarriage. ▶ Continued |

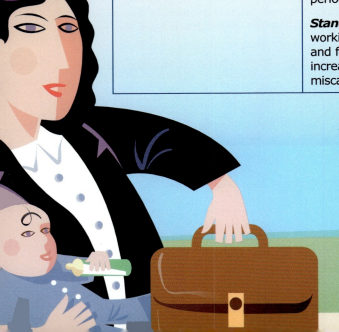

...nd 2 to the EC Directive on Pregnant Workers 92/85/EEC)[4]

| How to avoid the risk | Other legislation/guidance |
|---|---|
| ...ions and/or likely to disrupt placental attachment and in particular: | |
| Where appropriate, introduce or adapt work equipment and lifting gear, alter storage arrangements or redesign workstations or job content.

Pregnant women should avoid long periods spent handling loads, or standing or sitting without regular exercise or movement to maintain healthy circulation. You should provide the opportunity to alternate between standing and sitting. If this is not possible, you should provide for breaks. | Workplace (Health, Safety and Welfare) Regulations 1992 and Approved Code of Practice (ACOP)[2] cover the provision of suitable workstations and seating.

Health and Safety (Display Screen Equipment) Regulations 1992 and associated guidance[9] detail the factors you need to take into account to ensure that display screen equipment is safe and comfortable to use. |

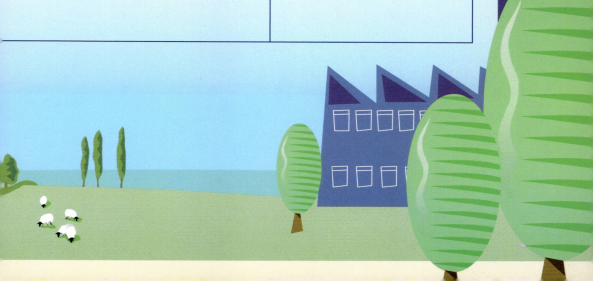

| List of agents/working conditions | What is the risk? |
|---|---|

## PHYSICAL RISKS *continued*

| | |
|---|---|
| **Movements and postures** *continued* | ***Sitting***: Pregnancy-specific changes pose a relatively high risk of thrombosis or embolism, particularly with constant sitting.  In the later stages of pregnancy, women are more likely to experience backache, which can be intensified by remaining in a specific position for a long period of time.<br><br>Backache in pregnancy may also be associated with prolonged work, poor working posture, and excessive movement.  A pregnant woman may need more workspace, or may need to adapt the way she works (or the way she interacts with the work of others or with her work equipment) as pregnancy changes both her size and the ways in which she can move, stand or sit still for a long time in comfort and safety.<br><br>***Confined space***: It is hazardous working in confined workspaces, or with workstations which do not adjust sufficiently to take account of increased abdominal size, particularly during the later stages of pregnancy.  This may lead to strain or sprain injuries.  Dexterity, agility, co-ordination, speed of movement, reach and balance may also be impaired and an increase in the risk of accidents may need to be considered. There may also be additional risks if a woman is returning to work after a childbirth with medical complications such as a Caesarean birth or deep vein thrombosis. |

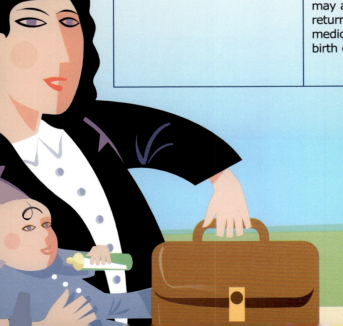

| List of agents/working conditions | What is the risk? |
|---|---|

## PHYSICAL RISKS *continued*

| | |
|---|---|
| **Manual handling of loads where there is a risk of injury** | Pregnant workers are especially at risk from manual handling injury. For example, hormonal changes can affect the ligaments, increasing susceptibility to injury; and postural problems may increase as the pregnancy progresses.<br><br>There can also be risks for those who have recently given birth. For example, after a Caesarean section there is likely to be a temporary limitation on lifting and handling capability.<br><br>Breastfeeding mothers may experience discomfort due to increased breast size and sensitivity. |
| **Shocks and vibration** | Regular exposure to shocks, low frequency vibration (for example driving or riding in off-road vehicles) or excessive movement may increase the risk of a miscarriage.<br><br>Long-term exposure to whole body vibration does not cause abnormalities to the unborn child.  However, there may be an increased risk of prematurity or low birth weight.<br><br>Breastfeeding workers are at no greater risk than other workers. |

| How to avoid the risk | Other legislation/guidance |
| --- | --- |
| The changes you should make will depend on the risks identified in the assessment and the circumstances of the business. For example, it may be possible to alter the nature of the task to reduce risks from manual handling for all workers including new or expectant mothers. Or you may have to address the specific needs of the worker and reduce the amount of physical work she does, or provide aids for her in future to reduce the risks she faces. | Manual Handling Operations Regulations 1992 require employers to: <br> ● avoid the need for hazardous manual handling, so far as is reasonably practicable; <br> ● assess the risks from those operations that cannot be avoided; and <br> ● take steps to reduce these risks to the lowest level reasonably practicable. <br><br> *Guidance on Regulations* [10] <br><br> *Getting to grips with manual handling – A short guide for employers*[11] |
| Pregnant workers and those who have recently given birth are advised to avoid work likely to involve uncomfortable whole body vibration, especially at low frequencies, or where the abdomen is exposed to shocks or jolts. | None specific. |

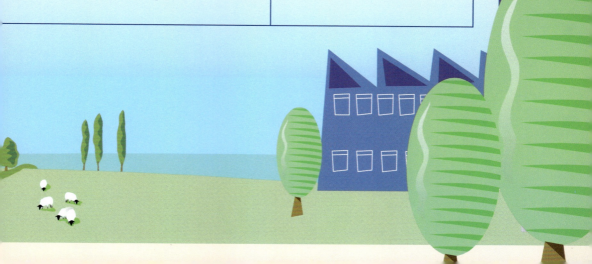

| List of agents/working conditions | What is the risk? |
|---|---|

**PHYSICAL RISKS** *continued*

| | |
|---|---|
| **Noise** | There appears to be no specific risk to new or expectant mothers, but prolonged exposure to loud noise may lead to increased blood pressure and tiredness.<br><br>No particular problems for women who have recently given birth or who are breastfeeding. |
| **Ionising radiation** | Significant exposure to ionising radiation can be harmful to the unborn child. You are required to ensure that the conditions of exposure during the remainder of the pregnancy are such that the dose to the unborn child is unlikely to exceed a value specified in the Ionising Radiations Regulations 1999.<br><br>The radiation hazard may arise from external sources. This can include cosmic radiation (radiation from the sun and from the galaxy), which increases with altitude and which may be relevant to aircraft crews and other frequent flyers. The radiation exposure to the abdomen of the expectant mother should be restricted.<br>▶ Continued |

| How to avoid the risk | Other legislation/guidance |
| --- | --- |
| The requirements of the Noise at Work Regulations 1989 should be sufficient to meet the needs of new or expectant mothers.<br><br>You must ensure that workers who are pregnant, who have recently given birth or who are breastfeeding are not exposed to noise levels exceeding national exposure limit values. | Noise at Work Regulations 1989 apply to all workers exposed to loud noise where there is a risk to hearing.<br><br>*Guidance on legislation*[12]<br><br>*Noise at work - advice for employers* [13] |
| Work procedures should be designed to keep exposure of the pregnant woman to a level which is as low as reasonably practicable (and so restrict the radiation dose to the unborn child to below that specified in the Ionising Radiation Regulations).<br><br>You must undertake a risk assessment. This should consider, depending upon specific working conditions, the risk from external radiation exposure to the abdomen of expectant mothers and possible contamination by or intake of radioactive materials by expectant mothers and breastfeeding women. | Ionising Radiations Regulations 1999 and supporting Approved Code of Practice[14]<br><br>*Working safely with ionising radiation: Guidelines for expectant or breastfeeding mothers* [15]<br><br>The Air Navigation Order 2000,[16] the Air Navigation (Cosmic Radiation) (Keeping of Records) Regulations 2000[17] and *Protection of air crew from cosmic radiation: guidance material*[18] issued by the Civil Aviation Authority. |

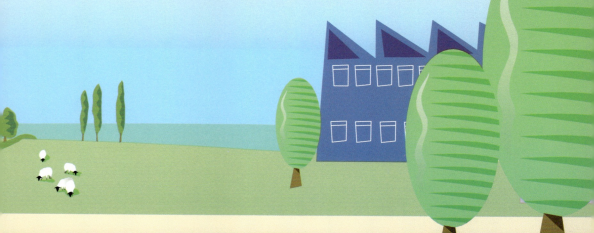

| List of agents/working conditions | What is the risk? |
|---|---|

## PHYSICAL RISKS *continued*

| | |
|---|---|
| **Ionising radiation** *continued* | If the work involves radioactive materials, there may be a risk to the unborn child if significant amounts are ingested or inhaled by the expectant mother or permeate through her skin and are transferred via the placenta to the unborn child. In addition, radiation from radioactive substances taken into the mother's body irradiates the unborn child through the wall of the womb.

Similarly, radioactive material may pass into the milk of a breastfeeding mother and therefore present a radiation hazard to the suckling infant.

Radioactive contamination of the skin of a nursing woman may also present a direct radiation hazard to the suckling infant. ■ |
| **Non-ionising electromagnetic radiation (NIEMR)** | ***Optical radiation***: pregnant or breastfeeding mothers are at no greater risk than other workers.

***Electromagnetic fields and waves*** (eg radio-frequency radiation): Exposure to electric and magnetic fields within current recommendations is not known to cause harm to the unborn child or the mother. However, extreme over-exposure to radio-frequency radiation could cause harm by raising body temperature. |

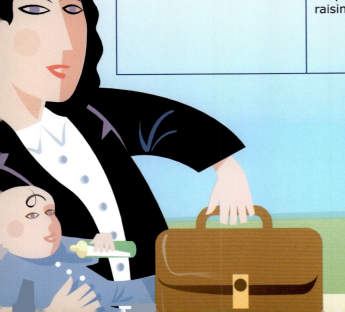

| How to avoid the risk | Other legislation/guidance |
|---|---|
| You must inform female workers who may be exposed to ionising radiation that they need to declare the pregnancy as soon as possible and to inform you if they are breastfeeding. You should also ensure that new and expectant mothers are given training, information and instruction to cover the fundamental and routine requirements in order to work with ionising radiation. | |
| Exposure to electric and magnetic fields should not exceed the restrictions on human exposure published by the National Radiological Protection Board.[19] | National Radiological Protection Board statement on restrictions on human exposure to static and time varying electromagnetic fields and radiation - 4, Nr5, 1993; pp1-63[19] |

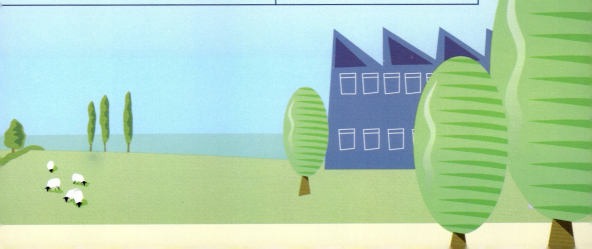

| List of agents/working conditions | What is the risk? |
|---|---|
| **PHYSICAL RISKS** *continued* | |
| **Work in hyperbaric atmosphere, for example pressurised enclosures and underwater diving** | *Compressed air*: People who work in compressed air are at risk of developing decompression illness (DCI), commonly known as the bends. This is due to free bubbles of gas in the circulation.<br><br>There is little scientific information whether pregnant women are at more risk of decompression illness but potentially the unborn child could be seriously harmed by such gas bubbles.<br><br>For those who have recently given birth there is a small increase in the risk of DCI.<br><br>There is no physiological reason why a breastfeeding mother should not work in compressed air (although there would be obvious practical difficulties).<br><br>*Diving*: Pregnant workers are advised not to dive *at all* during pregnancy due to the possible effects of exposure to a hyperbaric environment on the unborn child.<br><br>There is no evidence to suggest that breastfeeding and diving are incompatible |
| **Underground mining work** | Mines often have difficult physical conditions and many of the physical agents described in this guidance are a regular part of the mining environment. |

| How to avoid the risk | Other legislation/guidance |
|---|---|
| Pregnant workers should not work in compressed air. You should encourage workers to notify you (and Appointed Doctors under the Work in Compressed Air Regulations) as early as possible if they are pregnant. Women who are exposed to working in compressed air before the pregnancy is diagnosed should ensure that they tell their doctor and obstetrician at their routine antenatal appointments. | Work in Compressed Air Regulations 1996 and Approved Code of Practice[20] |
| Pregnancy is viewed as a medical reason not to dive. The diving regulations include the provision that if a diver knows of any medical reason why they should not dive, they should disclose it to the dive supervisor and/or refrain from diving.<br><br>The diving regulations also require all divers to undertake an annual medical examination. HSE advises doctors that pregnant workers should not dive. | The Diving at Work Regulations 1997[21] |
| Managers and contractors are responsible for assessing risks and should take action in line with suggestions elsewhere in this table. | |

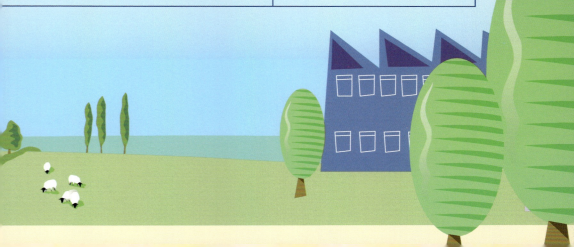

| List of agents/working conditions | What is the risk? |
|---|---|
| **BIOLOGICAL AGENTS** - infectious diseases | |
| **Any biological agent of hazard groups 2, 3 and 4 (Categorisation of biological agents according to hazard and categories of containment - Advisory Committee on Dangerous Pathogens)** | Many biological agents within these three risk groups can affect the unborn child if the mother is infected during pregnancy. These may be transmitted through the placenta while the child is in the womb, or during or after birth, for example through breastfeeding or through close physical contact between mother and child. Examples of agents where the child might be infected are hepatitis B, HIV (the AIDS virus), herpes, TB, syphilis, chickenpox and typhoid. For most workers, the risk of infection is not higher at work than from elsewhere, but in certain occupations exposure to infections is more likely, for example laboratory work, health care, looking after animals or dealing with animal products (eg meat processing). |
| **Biological agents known to cause abortion of the unborn child, or physical and neurological damage. These agents are included in hazard groups 2, 3 and 4.** | Rubella (German measles) and toxoplasma can harm the unborn child, as can some other biological agents, for example cytomegalovirus (an infection common outside the workplace) and chlamydia in sheep. The risks of infection are generally no higher for workers than for others except in exposed occupations (see above). |

| How to avoid the risk | Other legislation/guidance |
|---|---|
| This depends on the risk assessment, which will take account of the nature of the biological agent, how infection is spread, how likely contact is, and what control measures there are.<br><br>These control measures may include physical containment, hygiene measures, and using vaccines if exposure justifies this. If there is a known high risk of exposure to a highly infectious agent, then it will be appropriate for the pregnant worker to avoid exposure altogether.<br><br>Assessing the immunity of an employee in risk occupations can help you decide on their fitness for work and whether you need to take further steps to safeguard their health. However, testing for immunity is an invasive procedure and may not generally be appropriate. If you decide to assess immunity, you should only do this with the full consent of the individual. As with vaccination, you must provide information to the employee about immunity testing, including the perceived benefits and drawbacks. This will allow the individual to make an informed choice. | Control of Substances Hazardous to Health Regulations 1999<br><br>Approved Code of Practice on the control of biological agents[7]<br><br>*Infection risks to new and expectant mothers in the workplace - A guide for employers*[22] |
| See above.<br><br>The pregnant woman should avoid exposure to these biological agents unless she is protected by her state of immunity | See above. |

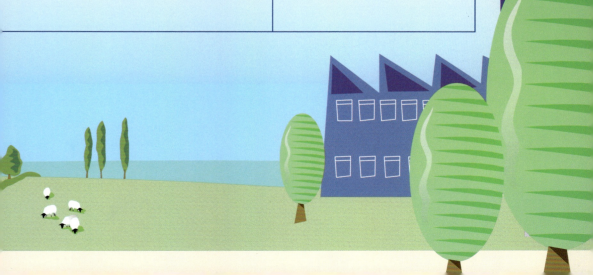

| List of agents/working conditions | What is the risk? |
| --- | --- |

**CHEMICAL AGENTS** - Chemical agents may enter the human body throu absorption. The following chemical agents insofar as it is known that th

| | |
| --- | --- |
| **Substances labelled R40, R45, R46, R49, R61, R63, R64 and R68** | There are a number of substances with hazardous properties indicated by these risk phrases, including about 1000 substances in the Approved Supply List:[23]<br>R40: limited evidence of a carcinogenic effect.<br>R45: may cause cancer.<br>R46: may cause heritable genetic damage.<br>R49: may cause cancer by inhalation.<br>R61: may cause harm to the unborn child.<br>R63: possible risk of harm to the unborn child.<br>R64: may cause harm to breastfed babies.<br>R68: possible risk of irreversible effects.<br><br>The actual risk to health of these substances can only be determined following a risk assessment of a particular substance at the place of work. Although the substances listed may have the potential to endanger health or safety, there may be no risk in practice, for example if exposure is at a level that is known to be safe. |

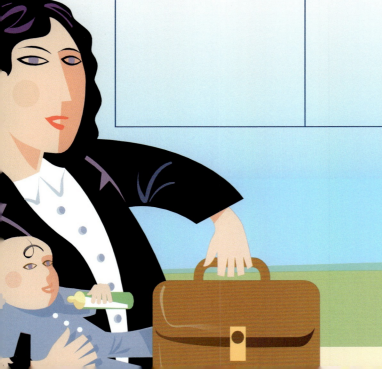

...ferent pathways: inhalation, ingestion, cuts and abrasions, and dermal ...danger the health of pregnant women and the unborn child:

| How to avoid the risk | Other legislation/guidance |
|---|---|
| For work with hazardous substances (which include chemicals which may cause heritable genetic damage) you are required to assess the health risks to workers arising from such work, and where appropriate prevent or control the risks. In carrying out assessments, you should have regard for women who are pregnant, or who have recently given birth. Occupational Exposure Limits (OELs) for workplace air are set under COSHH for specific substances, and reproductive toxicity is one of the health effects that is considered when setting limits. | With the exception of lead (see separate entry on lead on page 36) and asbestos these substances all fall within the scope of Control of Substances Hazardous to Health Regulations 1999 (COSHH)[7] and Chemicals (Hazard Information and Packaging for Supply) Regulations 2002 (CHIP).[23] |
| Preventing exposure must be your first priority. You should do this through substitution of harmful agents, if possible. | *COSHH: a brief guide to the regulations* [24] |
| Where it is not possible to eliminate exposure, you can control it by a combination of technical measures, along with good work planning and housekeeping, and the use of Personal Protective Equipment (PPE). You should only use PPE for control purposes if all other methods have failed. You may also use it as secondary protection in combination with other methods. | EH40 – *Occupational exposure limits*[25]  Interactive internet product www.coshh-essentials.org.uk |

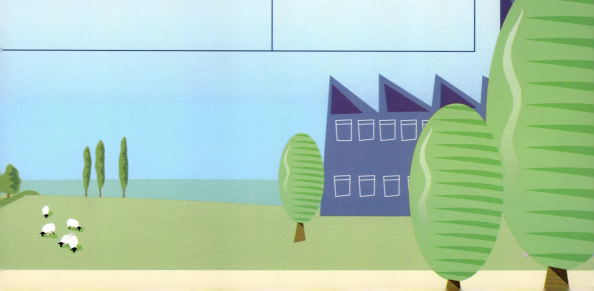

| List of agents/working conditions | What is the risk? |
|---|---|
| **CHEMICAL AGENTS** *continued* | |
| **Preparations labelled on the basis of Directive 1999/45/EC** | The principles outlined above should also be applied to preparations labelled with the risk phrases R40, R45, R46, R49, R61, R63, R64 or R68. |
| **Chemical agents and industrial processes in Annex 1 to Directive 90/394/EEC** | The substances, preparations and processes listed in Annex 1 of the EC Directive on the Control of Carcinogenic Substances are also covered by COSHH. |
| **Mercury and mercury derivatives** | Organic mercury compounds could have adverse effects on the unborn child. Animal studies and human observations have demonstrated that exposure to these forms of mercury during pregnancy can slow the growth of the unborn child, disrupt the nervous system, and poison the mother.<br><br>There is no clear evidence of adverse effects on the developing unborn child from studies of humans exposed to mercury and inorganic mercury compounds.<br><br>There is no indication that mothers are more likely to suffer greater adverse effects from mercury and its compounds after the birth of the baby.<br><br>Organic mercury can be transferred from blood to milk, therefore causing a potential risk to the newborn baby, if the mother is highly exposed before and during pregnancy. |

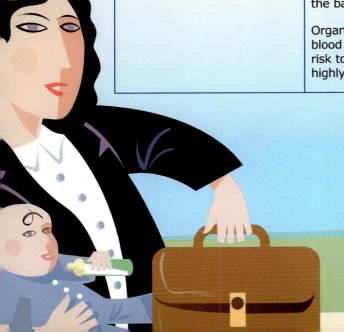

| How to avoid the risk | Other legislation/guidance |
|---|---|
|  |  |
| You should assess hazardous preparations and undertake risk management action in the same way as for similar hazardous substances. | COSHH[7] 1999<br><br>Chemical (Hazard Information and Packaging for Supply) Regulations 2002<br><br>*The idiot's guide to CHIP*[26] |
|  | COSHH[7] 1999 |
| Preventing exposure must be your first priority. Where it is not possible to eliminate exposure, you can control it by a combination of technical measures, along with good work planning and housekeeping, and the use of Personal Protective Equipment (PPE). You should only use PPE for control purposes if all other methods have failed. You may also use it as secondary protection in combination with other methods. | *Guidance notes Mercury and its inorganic divalent compounds*[27] and *Mercury - medical guidance notes*[28] give practical guidance on the risks of working with mercury and how to control them.<br><br>Mercury and mercury derivatives are covered by the requirements of COSHH. |

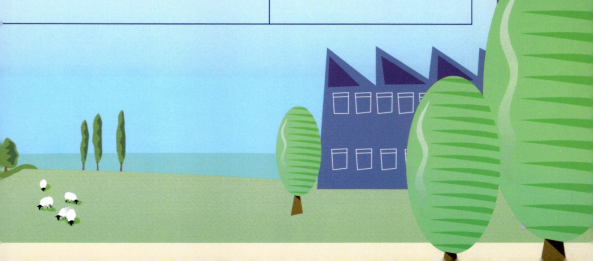

| List of agents/working conditions | What is the risk? |
|---|---|
| **CHEMICAL AGENTS** *continued* | |
| **Antimitotic (cytotoxic) drug** | In the long term these drugs cause damage to genetic information in sperm and eggs. Some can cause cancer. Absorption is by inhalation or through the skin. |

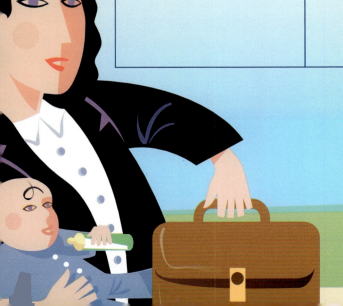

| How to avoid the risk | Other legislation/guidance |
|---|---|
| A safe level of exposure cannot be determined for these drugs, so you should avoid exposure or reduce it to as low a level as is reasonably practicable. | COSHH[7] 1999 |
| When assessing the risk you should look particularly at preparation of the drug for use (pharmacists and nurses), administration of the drug, and disposal of waste (chemical and human). | |
| All female employees of childbearing age should be fully informed of the reproductive hazard. | |
| When preparing the drug solutions, minimise exposure by using protective garments (gloves, gowns and masks), equipment (flow hood), and good working practices. A pregnant worker preparing antineoplastic drug solutions should be transferred to another job. | |

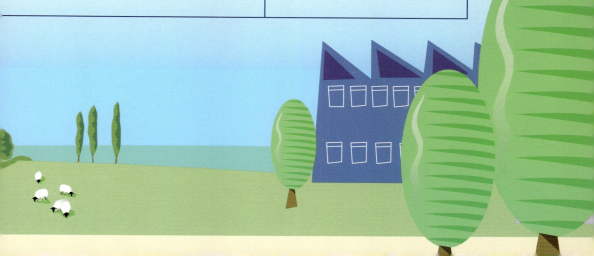

| List of agents/working conditions | What is the risk? |
| --- | --- |

## CHEMICAL AGENTS *continued*

**Chemical agents of known and dangerous percutaneous absorption (ie that may be absorbed through the skin). This includes some pesticides.**

The HSE guidance booklet EH40 *Occupational exposure limits*,[25] updated annually, contains tables of inhalation exposure limits for certain hazardous substances. Some of these substances can also penetrate intact skin and become absorbed into the body, causing ill-health effects. These substances are marked 'Sk' in the tables. As with all substances, the risks will depend on the way that the substance is being used as well as on its hazardous properties. Absorption through the skin can result from localised contamination, for example from a splash on the skin or clothing, or in certain cases from exposure to high atmospheric concentrations of vapour.

In the case of agricultural workers, the risk assessment should consider whether there is a residual risk of contamination, for example from exposure to pesticides at an earlier stage of pregnancy.

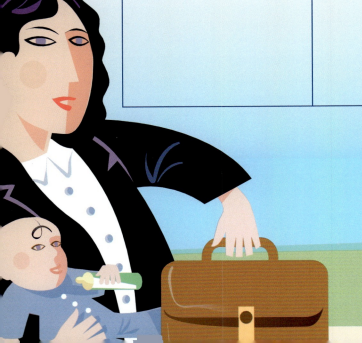

| How to avoid the risk | Other legislation/guidance |
| --- | --- |
| Preventing exposure must be your first priority. Take special precautions to prevent skin contact.<br><br>Where possible, use technical measures to control exposure in preference to personal protective equipment such as gloves, overalls or face shields. For example, enclose the process or redesign it so that less spray is produced. Where you must use personal protective equipment (either alone or in combination with engineering methods), ensure that it is suitable.<br><br>The Control of Pesticides Regulations sets out general restrictions on the way that pesticides can be used. In addition, all pesticides must be approved before they can be advertised, sold, supplied, used or stored. Conditions can be put onto the approval, which may for example limit the way the product can be used (eg restrict the way that it can be applied), require that certain safety precautions are followed, and restrict who may use it (eg professionals or amateurs). These conditions are reflected on the product label. Failure to comply is an offence. | COSHH[7] 1999<br><br>Control of Pesticides Regulations 1986 (COPR) |

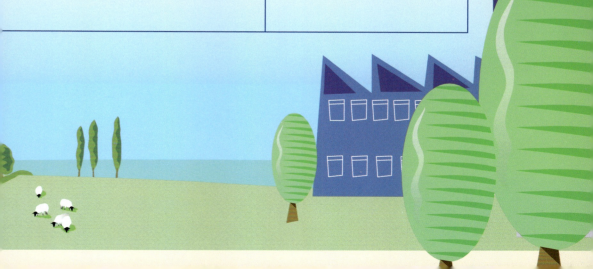

| List of agents/working conditions | What is the risk? |
| --- | --- |

## CHEMICAL AGENTS *continued*

**Carbon monoxide (CO)**

Carbon monoxide is produced when petrol, diesel and liquefied petroleum gas (LPG) are used as a source of power in engines and in domestic appliances. Risks arise when engines or appliances are operated in enclosed areas. Pregnant women may have heightened susceptibility to the effects of exposure to CO.

Carbon monoxide readily crosses the placenta and can result in the unborn child being starved of oxygen. Data on the effects of exposure to carbon monoxide on pregnant women are limited but there is evidence of adverse effects on the unborn child.

Both the level and duration of maternal exposure are important factors in the effect on the unborn child.

There is no indication that breastfed babies suffer adverse effects from their mothers' exposure to carbon monoxide, nor that mothers are significantly more sensitive to carbon monoxide after giving birth.

Given the extreme risk of exposure to high levels of carbon monoxide, risk assessment and prevention of high exposure are identical for all workers. Risk assessment may be complicated by active or passive smoking (see entry on passive smoking on page 46) or ambient air pollution. If those sources lead to a higher COHb (carbo-oxyhaemoglobin) than occupational exposure would, the level of risk is determined by those outside sources, as the effect on COHb is not cumulative.

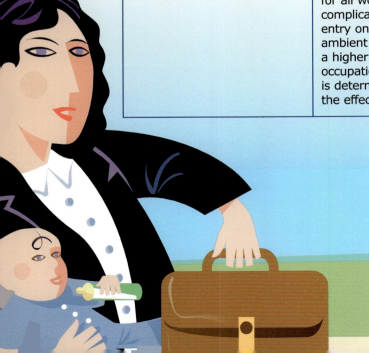

| How to avoid the risk | Other legislation/guidance |
|---|---|
| The best preventive measure is to eliminate the hazard by changing processes or equipment. Where prevention is not appropriate, you should consider technical measures, in combination with good working practices and personal protective equipment.<br><br>Avoid chronic exposure of female workers. Even occasional exposure to CO could potentially be harmful.<br><br>Inform pregnant workers about the dangers of exposure to carbon monoxide during smoking. | General requirements of COSHH[7] 1999 in relation to hazardous substances.<br><br>HSE's guidance note *Carbon monoxide*[29] gives practical advice on the risks of working with carbon monoxide and how to control them. It warns that pregnant women may have heightened susceptibility to the effects of exposure to carbon monoxide. |

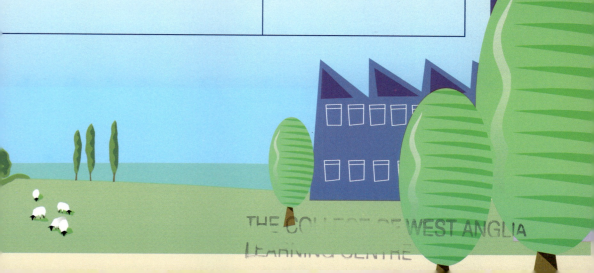

| List of agents/working conditions | What is the risk? |
|---|---|

### CHEMICAL AGENTS *continued*

**Lead and lead derivatives - insofar as these agents are capable of being absorbed by the human organism**

Historically, exposure to lead by pregnant women has been associated with abortions, miscarriages, stillbirths, and infertility. However, there is no indication that this is still relevant at current accepted standards for exposure. There are strong indications that exposure to lead, either before or after birth via the mother or during early childhood, can impair the development of the child's nervous system.

Lead can be transferred from blood to milk. This may pose a risk to the newborn baby, if the mother has been highly exposed before and during pregnancy.

***Indications of safe levels***
Exposure to lead cannot safely be accurately determined by the measurements of the airborne concentration because uptake from the oral route may also occur and because of differences in the uptake characteristics of the various forms of lead that may be encountered. Biological monitoring of blood lead levels (PbB) and biological effects monitoring (eg tests for zinc proto porphyrin and levels of amino laevulinic acid in blood or urine) are the best exposure indicator.

***Risk assessment***
The exposure of pregnant and breastfeeding women to lead is specifically prohibited under Article 6 of the Directive (92/85/EEC) if the exposure might jeopardise safety or health.
Continued ▶

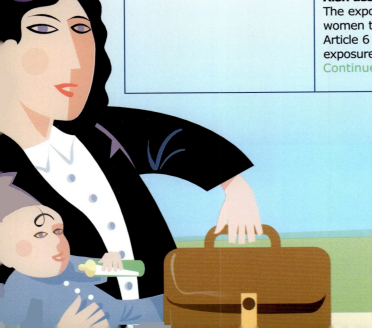

| How to avoid the risk | Other legislation/guidance |
|---|---|
| The Approved Code of Practice *Control of lead at work*[36] sets out the current exposure limits for lead and the blood-lead suspension levels for workers whose exposure to lead is significant and subject to medical surveillance. It gives a blood-lead suspension level for male adults and for women who cannot conceive, a lower level for young persons under 18 and a lower level still for women of reproductive capacity. This lowest level is set to ensure that women who may become pregnant have low blood lead levels. This is to protect any developing foetus from the harmful effects of lead in the weeks before a pregnancy is confirmed.<br><br>Once their pregnancy is confirmed, women will normally be suspended from any work which exposes them significantly to lead, by the Employment Medical Adviser or Appointed Doctor carrying out the medical surveillance. | Control of Lead at Work Regulations 1999 (CLAW) and Approved Code of Practice[6] |

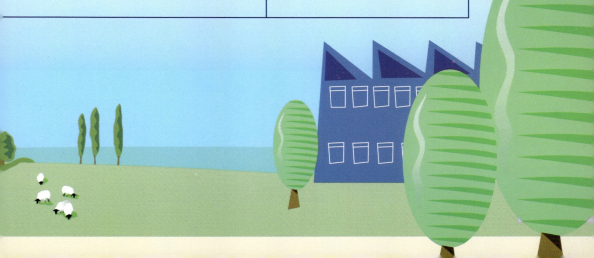

| List of agents/working conditions | What is the risk? |
|---|---|

**CHEMICAL AGENTS** *continued*

**Lead and lead derivatives** *continued*

The risk assessment should be based upon both the individual's and the work group's historical record of blood lead levels or similar parameters, not on ambient air monitoring. Where these are within the range found in people not occupationally exposed to lead, it could be concluded that the health is not in jeopardy. However, PbB levels and other biological indicators of exposure may change over time without apparent relation to (airborne) exposure. ▪

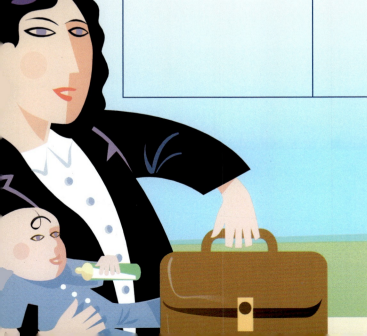

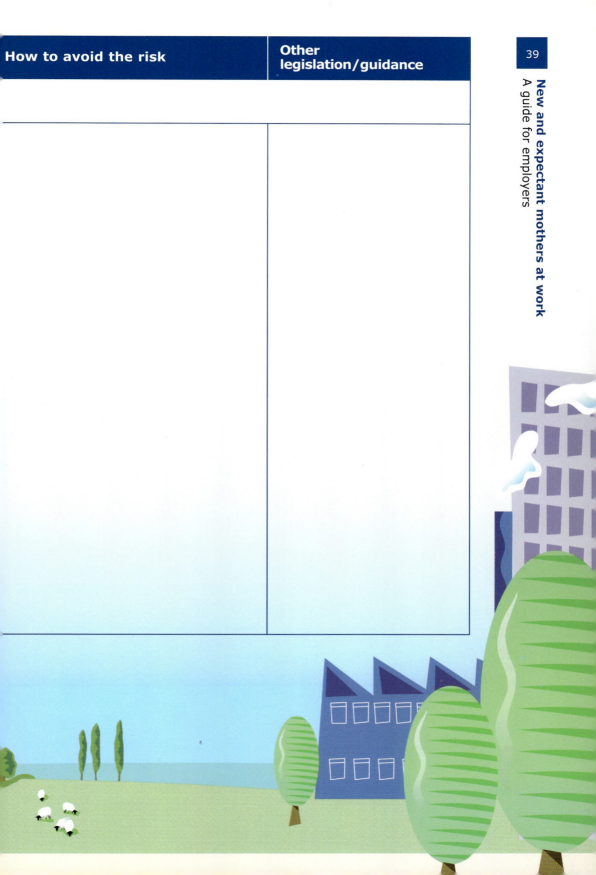

| List of agents/working conditions | What is the risk? |
|---|---|

## WORKING CONDITIONS

**Facilities**

*Resting facilities*: Rest is important for new and expectant mothers. Tiredness increases during and after pregnancy and may be exacerbated by work-related factors. The need for rest is both physical and mental.

*Hygiene facilities*: Without easy access to toilets (and associated hygiene facilities) at work, due to distance, work processes or systems, etc, there may be increased risks to health and safety, including significant risks of infection and kidney disease.

Because of pressure on the bladder and other changes associated with pregnancy, pregnant women often have to go to the toilet more frequently and more urgently than others. Breastfeeding women may also need to do so because of increased fluid intake to promote breast milk production.

*Storage facilities*: Access to appropriate facilities for breastfeeding mothers to express and safely store breast milk, or to enable infants to be breastfed at or near the workplace, may facilitate breastfeeding by working women, and may significantly protect the health of both mother and infant.

Evidence shows that breastfeeding can help to protect the mother against cancer and helps protect the child from certain diseases in infancy. Obstacles to breastfeeding in the workplace may significantly affect the health of both mother and child.

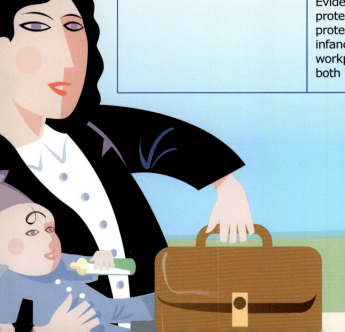

The need for physical rest may require that the woman concerned has access to somewhere where she can sit or lie down comfortably in privacy, and without disturbance, at appropriate intervals. Access to clean drinking water should also be available.

Protective measures include adapting rules governing working practices, for example in continuous processing and teamworking situations, and appropriate measures to enable expectant and nursing mothers to leave their workstation/activity at short notice more frequently than normal, or otherwise (if this is not possible) making temporary adjustments to working conditions as specified in the Management of Health and Safety at Work Regulations.

Protective measures include:
- access to a private room where women can breastfeed or express breast milk;
- use of secure, clean refrigerators for storing expressed breast milk while at work, and facilities for washing, sterilising and storing receptacles;
- time off (without loss of pay or benefits, and without fear of penalty) to express milk or breastfeed.

Workplace (Health, Safety and Welfare) Regulations 1992 and Approved Code of Practice[2] cover the need to provide suitable and sufficient rest facilities.

Management of Health and Safety at Work Regulations 1999 and Approved Code of Practice[1]

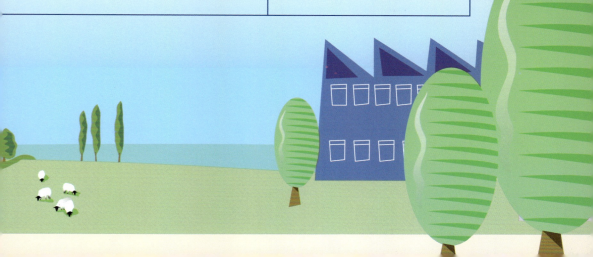

| List of agents/working conditions | What is the risk? |
| --- | --- |

## WORKING CONDITIONS *continued*

| | |
| --- | --- |
| **Mental and physical fatigue and working hours** | Long working hours, shift work and night work can have a significant effect on the health of new and expectant mothers, and on breastfeeding. Not all women are affected in the same way, and the associated risks vary with the type of work undertaken, the working conditions and the individual concerned. This applies especially to health care. Generally, however, both mental and physical fatigue increases during pregnancy and in the postnatal period due to the various physiological and other changes taking place.

Because they suffer from increasing tiredness, some pregnant and breastfeeding women may not be able to work irregular or late shifts or night work, or overtime. Working time arrangements (including provisions for rest breaks, and their frequency and timing) may affect the health of the pregnant woman and her unborn child, her recovery after childbirth, or her ability to breastfeed, and may increase the risks of stress and stress-related ill health. Because of changes in blood pressure which may occur during and after pregnancy and childbirth, normal patterns of breaks from work may not be adequate for new or expectant mothers. |

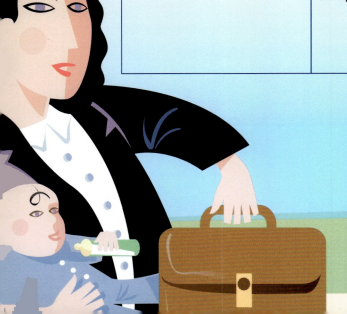

| How to avoid the risk | Other legislation/guidance |
|---|---|
| It may be necessary to adjust working hours temporarily, as well as other working conditions, including the timing and frequency of rest breaks, and to change shift patterns and duration to avoid risks.<br><br>With regard to night work, alternative day work should be organised for pregnant women on receipt of a medical certificate from their doctor/midwife which states that night work is affecting the health and safety of the woman or her unborn child. | Workplace (Health, Safety and Welfare) Regulations 1992 and Approved Code of Practice[2] |

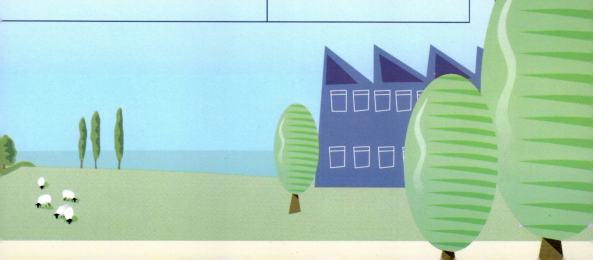

| List of agents/working conditions | What is the risk? |
|---|---|

## WORKING CONDITIONS *continued*

| **Occupational stress** | New and expectant mothers can be particularly vulnerable to occupational stressors, for various reasons: |
|---|---|

- Hormonal, physiological and psychological changes occur and sometimes change rapidly during and after pregnancy, sometimes affecting susceptibility to stress, or to anxiety or depression in individuals.
- Financial, emotional and job insecurity may be issues, due to changes in economic circumstances brought about by pregnancy, especially if this is reflected in workplace culture.
- It may be difficult to organise work and private life, especially with long, unpredictable or unsociable working hours or where other family responsibilities are involved.

Additional stress may occur if a woman's anxiety about her pregnancy, or about its outcome (eg where there is a past history of miscarriage, stillbirth or other abnormality) is heightened as a result of peer group or other pressure in the workplace. This can lead to increased vulnerability to other organisational stressors.

Stress is associated in some studies with increased incidence of miscarriage and pregnancy loss, and also with impaired ability to breastfeed. ▶ Continued

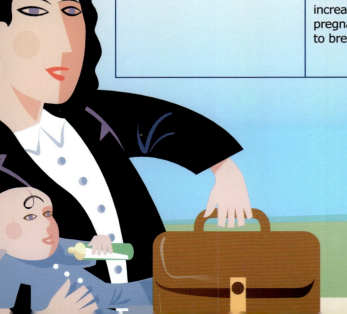

You will need to take account of known organisational stress factors (such as shift patterns, job insecurity, workloads, etc) and the particular medical and psychosocial factors affecting the individual woman.

Protective measures may include adjustments to working conditions or working hours, and ensuring that the necessary understanding, support and recognition is available when the woman returns to work, while her privacy is also respected.

*Tackling work-related stress. A manager's guide to improving and maintaining employee health and well-being*[30]

*Work-related stress. A short guide*[31]

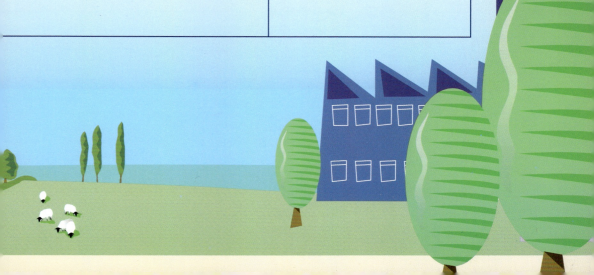

| List of agents/working conditions | What is the risk? |
|---|---|

### WORKING CONDITIONS *continued*

| | |
|---|---|
| **Occupational stress** *continued* | Women who have recently suffered loss through stillbirth, miscarriage, adoption at birth or neonatal death will be especially vulnerable to stress, as will women who have experienced serious illness or trauma (including Caesarean section) associated with pregnancy or childbirth. However, in some circumstances, returning to work after such events may help to alleviate stress, but only in those cases where there is a sympathetic and supportive work environment.<br><br>It is known that stress at work can lead to anxiety and depression. Conversely, if someone is already suffering from anxiety or depression, they may be more vulnerable to stressors in the workplace and therefore more likely to experience work-related stress. As such, it is important that managers remember that some women may develop postnatal depression after childbirth, which could make them more vulnerable to stressors. ■ |
| **Passive smoking** | Cigarette smoke is mutagenic and carcinogenic and is a known risk to pregnancy where the mother smokes. Cigarette smoke can also aggravate preconditions such as asthma. The effects of passive smoking are less clear but are known to affect the heart and lungs, and to pose a risk to infant health. |

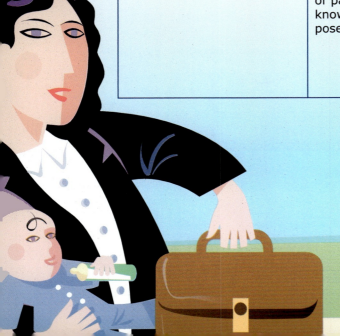

| How to avoid the risk | Other legislation/guidance |
|---|---|
| You should draw up a smoking policy which gives priority to the needs of non-smokers.<br><br>You should arrange rest areas and rest rooms to enable employees to use them without experiencing discomfort from tobacco smoke. This means that either smoking should be banned in them or separate smoking and non-smoking rooms/areas should be provided. | Workplace (Health, Safety and Welfare) Regulations 1992 and Approved Code of Practice[2]<br><br>*Passive smoking at work*[32] |

| List of agents/working conditions | What is the risk? |
|---|---|

## WORKING CONDITIONS *continued*

| | |
|---|---|
| **Extremes of cold or heat** | Prolonged exposure of pregnant workers to hot environments should be kept to a minimum, as there is a greater risk of the worker suffering from heat stress.<br><br>Working in extreme cold may be a hazard for pregnant women and their unborn children. Warm clothing should be provided.<br><br>The risks are particularly increased if there are sudden changes in temperature.<br><br>Breastfeeding may be impaired by heat dehydration. |
| **Work with display screen equipment (VDUs)** | Although it is not specifically listed in the Directive (92/85/EEC),[4] HSE is aware that anxiety about radiation emissions from display screen equipment and possible effects on pregnant women used to be widespread. However, there is substantial evidence that these concerns are unfounded. HSE has consulted the National Radiological Protection Board, which has the statutory function of providing information and advice on all radiation matters to Government departments, and the advice below summarises scientific understanding:<br><br>The levels of ionising and non-ionising electromagnetic radiation which are likely to be generated by display screen equipment  ► Continued |

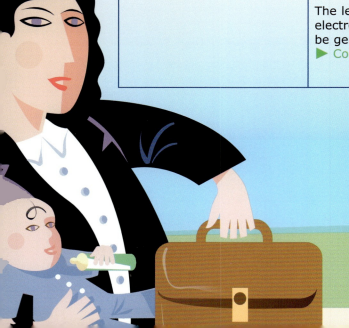

| How to avoid the risk | Other legislation/guidance |
|---|---|
| You should provide adequate rest and refreshment breaks alongside unrestricted access to drinking water.<br><br>New and expectant mothers should note that thirst is not an early indicator of heat stress. They should drink water before they get thirsty, preferably in small and frequent volumes. | |
| In light of the scientific evidence pregnant women do not need to stop work with VDUs. However, to avoid problems caused by stress and anxiety, women who are pregnant or planning children and worried about working with VDUs should be given the opportunity to discuss their concerns with someone adequately informed of current authoritative scientific information and advice. | Health and Safety (Display Screen Equipment) Regulations 1992[9] |

| List of agents/working conditions | What is the risk? |
|---|---|

## WORKING CONDITIONS *continued*

| | |
|---|---|
| **Work with display screen equipment (VDUs)** *continued* | are well below those set out in international recommendations for limiting risk to human health created by such emissions and the National Radiological Protection Board does not consider such levels to pose a significant risk to health. No special protective measures are therefore needed to protect the health of people from this radiation (see also the entry on physical agents on page 12).

There has been considerable public concern about reports of higher levels of miscarriage and birth defects among some groups of visual display unit (VDU) workers, in particular due to electromagnetic radiation. Many scientific studies have been carried out, but taken as a whole their results do not show any link between miscarriages or birth defects and working with VDUs. Research and reviews of the scientific evidence will continue to be undertaken. ▮ |
| **Working alone** | Pregnant women are more likely to need urgent medical attention. |

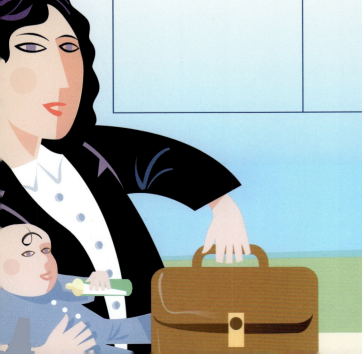

| How to avoid the risk | Other legislation/guidance |
|---|---|
| | |
| Depending on their medical condition, you may need to review and revise women's access to communications with others and levels of (remote) supervision involved, to ensure that help and support is available when required, and that emergency procedures (if needed) take into account the needs of new and expectant mothers. | *Working alone in safety: Controlling the risks of solitary work*[33] |

| List of agents/working conditions | What is the risk? |
|---|---|
| **WORKING CONDITIONS** *continued* | |
| **Work at heights** | It is hazardous for pregnant women to work at heights, for example ladders, platforms. |
| **Travelling either inside or outside the workplace** | Travelling in the course of work, and to and from the workplace, can be problematic for pregnant women, involving risks including fatigue, vibrations, stress, static posture, discomfort and accidents. These risks can have a significant effect on the health of new and expectant mothers. |
| **Work-related violence** | If a woman is exposed to the risk of violence at work during pregnancy, when she has recently given birth or while she is breastfeeding this may be harmful. It can lead to detachment of the placenta, miscarriage, premature delivery and underweight birth, and it may affect the ability to breastfeed.<br><br>This risk particularly affects workers in direct contact with customers and clients. |

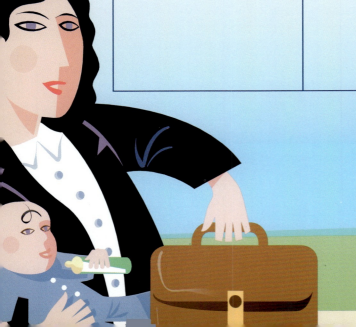

| How to avoid the risk | Other legislation/guidance |
|---|---|
| | |
| A risk assessment should consider any additional risks due to work at height (eg working on ladders). | |
| See specific entries in this table to assess how to reduce risk from fatigue, vibrations, stress, static posture etc. | |
| Measures to reduce the risk of violence include:<br>• providing adequate training and information for staff;<br>• improving the design or layout of the workplace;<br>• changing the design of the job - eg avoiding lone working, reducing use of cash, maintaining contact with workers away from work base.<br><br>If you cannot significantly reduce the risk of violence you should offer pregnant women and new mothers suitable alternative work. | Management of Health and Safety at Work Regulations 1999 and Approved Code of Practice[1]<br><br>*Violence at work: A guide for employers*[34]<br><br>Sector-specific guidance for health services,[35] education,[36] retail,[37] and banks and building societies[38] |

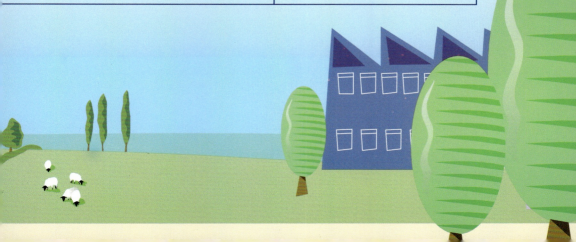

| List of agents/working conditions | What is the risk? |
|---|---|

## WORKING CONDITIONS *continued*

| | |
|---|---|
| **Work equipment and personal protective equipment (including clothing)** | Work equipment and personal protective equipment is not generally designed for use by pregnant women. Pregnancy (and breastfeeding) involves physiological changes which may make some existing work and protective equipment not only uncomfortable but also unsafe for use in some cases - for example, where equipment does not fit properly or comfortably, or where the operational mobility, dexterity or co-ordination of the woman concerned is temporarily impeded by her pregnancy or recent childbirth. |
| **Hazards as a result of inappropriate nutrition** | Adequate and appropriate nutrition and liquid refreshment (especially clean drinking water) at regular intervals is essential to the health of the new or expectant mother and her child(ren). Appetite and digestion are affected by the timing, frequency and duration of meal breaks and other opportunities for eating and drinking, and this also affects the health of the unborn child. This is affected during and after pregnancy by hormonal and physiological changes, including those resulting in or affecting 'morning' sickness (usually in early pregnancy), the position of the unborn child in the womb, the nutritional needs of the individual mother and her unborn or breastfeeding child(ren), etc. <br> ▶ Continued |

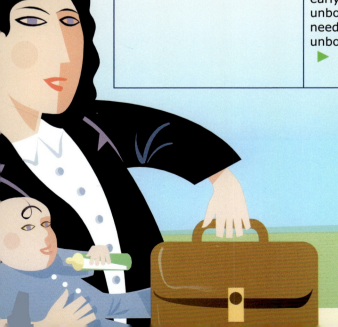

| How to avoid the risk | Other legislation/guidance |
|---|---|
| You must carry out a risk assessment which takes account of changes in risks as pregnancy progresses.<br><br>Wherever possible, the risk should be avoided by adaptations or substitution, eg providing suitable alternative equipment to allow the work to be conducted safely and without risk to health. Where this is not possible, the provisions of the Management of Health and Safety at Work Regulations come into effect. You must not allow unsafe working. | Management of Health and Safety at Work Regulations 1999 and Approved Code of Practice[1]<br><br>*Safe use of work equipment* Approved Code of Practice[39]<br><br>Personal Protective Equipment at Work Regulations 1992 and Guidance on Regulations[40] |
| You can establish new and expectant mothers' particular needs concerning rest, meal and refreshment breaks by consulting the individuals concerned. These needs may change as the pregnancy progresses.<br><br>You must take protective measures to deal with these constraints, particularly with regard to the need for rest, meal and refreshment breaks, and to maintain appropriate hygiene standards. | Workplace (Health, Safety and Welfare) Regulations and Approved Code of Practice[2] cover provision of welfare facilities |

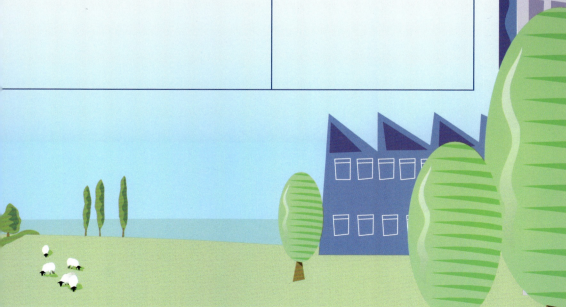

| List of agents/working conditions | What is the risk? |
|---|---|

## WORKING CONDITIONS *continued*

| | |
|---|---|
| **Hazards as a result of inappropriate nutrition** *continued* | Pregnant women may need more frequent meal breaks and more frequent access to drinking water or other light refreshments. They may also only be able to tolerate food 'little and often' rather than in larger quantities at 'normal' mealtimes. Their eating patterns and preferences may change, especially in early stages of pregnancy, not only in response to 'morning' sickness but also due to discomfort or other problems in the later stages of pregnancy. ■ |

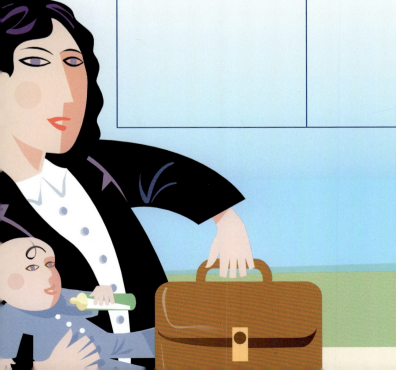

# Appendix 2
# Aspects of pregnancy which may affect work

Apart from the hazards listed in Appendix 1, there are other aspects of pregnancy that may affect work. The impact will vary during the course of the pregnancy and you will want to keep their effects under review, for example the posture of expectant mothers changes to cope with increasing size.

| Aspects of pregnancy | Factors in work |
| --- | --- |
| 'Morning' sickness<br>Headaches | Early shift work<br>Exposure to nauseating smells |
| Backache | Standing/manual handling/posture |
| Varicose veins | Standing/sitting |
| Haemorrhoids | Working in hot conditions |
| Frequent visits to toilet | Difficulty in leaving job/site of work |
| Increasing size | Use of protective clothing<br>Work in confined areas<br>Manual handling |
| Tiredness | Overtime<br>Evening work |
| Balance | Problems of working on slippery, wet surfaces |
| Comfort | Problems of working in tightly fitting work uniforms |

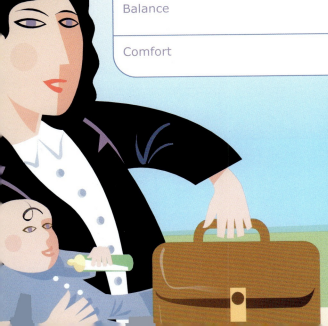

# Appendix 3
# Other legislation

1 The general duties outlined earlier in this guidance explained the requirements of the Management of Health and Safety at Work Regulations[1] and the Workplace (Health, Safety and Welfare) Regulations.[2] Appendix 1 set out possible hazards and other relevant regulations that apply.

2 The following legislation also places requirements on you to ensure the health and safety of new and expectant mothers and that of their children.

## Employment Rights Act 1996[41]

3 If action 1 (see figure one) is not reasonable or would not avoid the risk, a new or expectant mother has a right to be offered suitable alternative work, if any is available. The work must be:

- both suitable and appropriate for her to do in the circumstances; and
- on terms and conditions no less favourable than her normal terms and conditions.

4 An employee is entitled to make a complaint to an Employment Tribunal if there is suitable alternative work available which her employer has failed to offer to her before suspending her from work on maternity grounds.

5 If an employee has a medical certificate stating that night work could affect her health or safety, she has a right to be offered suitable alternative daytime work on terms and conditions no less favourable than her normal terms and conditions.

6 An employee suspended from work on these grounds is entitled to be paid remuneration (wages or salary) at her full normal rate for as long as the suspension continues. The only exception is where she has unreasonably refused an offer of suitable alternative work, in which case no remuneration is payable for the period during which the offer applies. If an employee has both statutory and a contractual rights to remuneration during maternity suspension, these entitlements can be offset against each other.

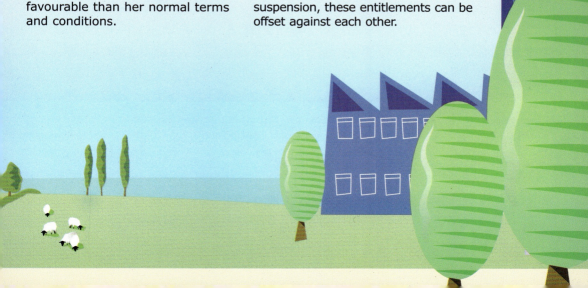

7 The employee continues to be employed during the maternity suspension period, so this counts towards her period of continuous employment for the purposes of assessing seniority, pension rights, and other personal length-of-service payments, such as pay increments. However, there is no statutory requirement for contractual benefits apart from remuneration to be continued during the maternity suspension itself. This, like most other terms and conditions of employment, remains a matter for negotiation and agreement on a voluntary or contractual basis between the parties concerned. You should however ensure that you are not acting unlawfully under the Equal Pay Act 1970[42] and the Sex Discrimination Act 1975.[43]

8 If you fail to pay your employee some or all of the remuneration due for any day of maternity suspension she is entitled to make a complaint to an Employment Tribunal.

# The Sex Discrimination Act 1975[43]

9 This Act makes it unlawful to discriminate on the ground of gender and married status in employment. The Act has no length of service qualification and gives protective rights to a broad range of workers including the self-employed, agency workers, apprentices, and voluntary workers, depending on the nature of their contract.

10 It has been established in law that discrimination that is substantially because of a woman's pregnancy is automatically unlawful sex discrimination. This principle has been extended to include the failure to conduct a risk assessment for women under the health and safety regulations. Women who have experienced a detriment arising from a failure to comply with these health and safety regulations can bring a tribunal claim under the Sex Discrimination Act, as well as exercising their rights under the Employment Rights Act.

11 The Sex Discrimination Act also makes an individual employee liable for their own actions and you are liable for unlawful actions of your employees, even where they are done without your knowledge or approval.

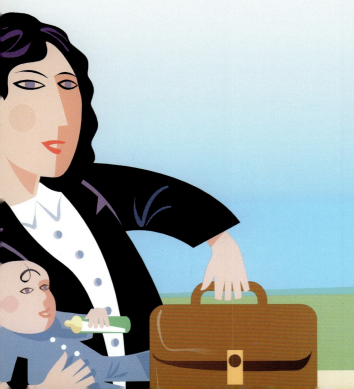

This means that an organisation needs to:

- have an adequate procedure specifying the particular steps to be followed, which clearly sets out individual responsibilities and enables complaints and concerns to be addressed quickly and efficiently;
- train employees and other workers on the regulations and the organisation's policy and procedures;
- regularly review how the procedures are being applied, and revise them as appropriate; and
- take appropriate action where managers/supervisors fail to implement the regulations appropriately.

The full text of The Sex Discrimination Act 1975 is available on the Equal Opportunities Commission's website: www.eoc.org.uk

# Further information
# References

1 *Management of health and safety at work. Management of Health and Safety at Work Regulations 1999. Approved Code of Practice and guidance* L21 (Second edition) HSE Books 2000 ISBN 0 7176 2488 9

2 *Workplace health, safety and welfare. Workplace (Health, Safety and Welfare) Regulations 1992. Approved Code of Practice* L24 HSE Books 1992 ISBN 0 7176 0413 6

3 *Five steps to risk assessment* INDG163 (rev1) HSE Books 1997

4 European Directive on the health and safety of pregnant workers 92/85/EEC European Commission Official Journal L348 28/11/1992

5 *Guidelines on the assessment of chemical, physical and biological agents and industrial processes considered hazardous for the safety or health of pregnant workers, workers who have recently given birth or are breastfeeding* European Commission 2000 COM(2000) 466Final/2.

6 *Control of lead at work. Control of Lead at Work Regulations 1998. Management of Health and Safety at Work Regulations 1992.*

*Workplace (Health, Safety and Welfare) Regulations 1992. Approved Code of Practice, Regulations and guidance* COP2 (Second edition) HSE Books 1998 ISBN 0 7176 1506 5 (this is expected to be revised in 2002/03)

7 *General COSHH ACOP (Control of substances hazardous to health) and Carcinogens ACOP (Control of carcinogenic substances) and Biological agents ACOP (Control of biological agents). Control of Substances Hazardous to Health Regulations 1999. Approved Codes of Practice* L5 (Third edition) HSE Books 1999 ISBN 0 7176 1670 3 (this is expected to be revised in 2002/03)

8 DTI *Maternity rights – A guide for employers and employees* URN 99/1191

9 *Display screen equipment work. Health and Safety (Display Screen Equipment) Regulations 1992. Guidance on Regulations* L26 HSE Books 1992 ISBN 07176 0410 1

10 *Manual handling. Manual Handling Operations Regulations 1992. Guidance on Regulations* L23 HSE Books 1998 ISBN 0 7176 2415 3

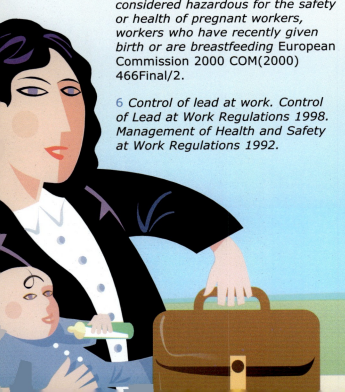

11 *Getting to grips with manual handling. A short guide for employers* INDG14 (rev1) HSE Books 2000

12 *Reducing noise at work. Guidance on Noise at Work Regulations* 1989 L108 HSE Books 1998 0 7176 1511 1

13 *Noise at work - advice for employers* INDG 362 HSE Books 2002

14 *Work with ionising radiation. Ionising Radiations Regulations 1999. Approved Code of Practice and guidance* L121 HSE Books 2000 ISBN 0 7176 1746 7

15 *Working safely with ionising radiation. Guidelines for expectant or breastfeeding mothers* INDG334 HSE Books 2001

16 *The Air Navigation Order 2000* SI 2000/1562 The Stationery Office 2000 ISBN 0 11 099408 6

17 *The Air Navigation (Cosmic Radiation) (Keeping of Records) Regulations 2000* SI 2000/1380 The Stationery Office 2000 ISBN 0 11 099341 1

18 Civil Aviation Authority *Protection of air crew from cosmic radiation: guidance material* Available online at www.caa.co.uk/docs/49/srg_med_co smicradiation.pdf

19 *Restrictions on human exposure to static and time varying electromagnetic fields and radiations* Documents of the NRPB 1993, vol 4, no 5 National Radiological Protection Board 1993 ISBN 0859513661

20 *A guide to the Work in Compressed Air Regulations 1996. Guidance on Regulations* L96 HSE Books 1996 ISBN 07176 1120 5

21 *The Diving at Work Regulations 1997* SI 1997/2776 The Stationery Office 1997 ISBN 0 11 0651707

22 *Infection risks to new and expectant mothers in the workplace: A guide for employers* Guidance booklet HSE Books 1997 ISBN 0 7176 1360 7

23 *Approved supply list (seventh edition). Information approved for the classification and labelling of substances and preparations dangerous for supply. Chemicals (Hazard Information and Packaging for Supply) Regulations 2002. Approved list* L129 (Seventh edition) HSE Books 2002 ISBN 0 7176 2368 8

24 *COSHH: a brief guide to the regulations. What you need to know about the Control of Substances Hazardous to Health Regulations 1999* (COSHH) INDG136 (rev 1) HSE Books 1999 Single copies free, priced packs of 10 ISBN 0 7176 2444 7 (this is expected to be revised in 2003)

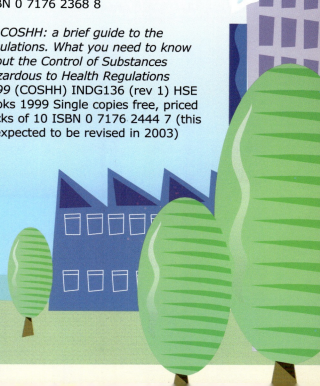

25 *Occupational exposure limits: Containing the list of maximum exposure limits and occupational exposure standards for use with the Control of Substances Hazardous to Health Regulations 1999* Guidance Note EH40 (revised annually) HSE Books 2001 Environmental Hygiene ISBN 0 7176 2083 2

26 *The idiot's guide to CHIP: Chemicals (Hazard Information and Packaging for Supply) Regulations 2002* Leaflet INDG350 HSE Books 2002 (single copy free or priced packs of 5 ISBN 0 7176 2333 5)

27 *Mercury and its inorganic divalent compounds* Environmental Hygiene Guidance Note EH17 (Second edition) HSE Books 1996 ISBN 0 7176 1127 2

28 *Mercury: Medical guidance notes* Medical Guidance Note MS12 (Second edition) HSE Books 1996 0 7176 1252 X

29 *Carbon monoxide: Health hazards and precautionary measures* Environmental Guidance Note EH43 (Second edition) HSE Books 1998 ISBN 0 7176 1501 4

30 *Tackling work-related stress. A manager's guide to improving and maintaining employee health and well-being* HSG218 HSE Books 2001 ISBN 0 7176 2050 6

31 *Work-related stress. A short guide* INDG281 (rev1) HSE Books 2001

32 *Passive smoking at work* INDG63 (rev1) HSE Books 1992

33 *Working alone in safety: Controlling the risks of solitary work* Leaflet INDG73 (rev) HSE Books 1998 (single copy free or priced packs of 15 ISBN 0 7176 1507 3)

34 *Violence at work. A guide for employers* INDG69 (rev) HSE Books 1996

35 *Violence and aggression to staff in health services: Guidance on assessment and management* (Second edition) Guidance Booklet HSE Books 1997 ISBN 0 7176 1466 2

36 *Violence in the education sector* (Second edition) Guidance Booklet HSE Books 1997 ISBN 0 7176 1293 7

37 *Preventing violence to retail staff* HSG133 HSE Books 1995 ISBN 0 7176 0891 3

38 *Prevention of violence to staff in banks and building societies* HSG100 HSE Books 1993 ISBN 0 7176 0683 X

39 *Safe use of work equipment. Provision and use of Work Equipment Regulations 1998. Approved Code of Practice and guidance* L22 (Second edition) HSE Books 1998 ISBN 0 7176 1626 6

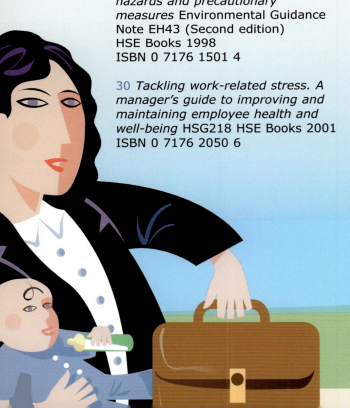

40 *Personal protective equipment at work. Personal Protective Equipment at Work Regulations 1992. Guidance on Regulations* L25 HSE Books 1992 ISBN 0 7176 0415 2

41 *The Employment Rights Act 1996* The Stationery Office ISBN 0 10 541896 X

42 *The Equal Pay Act 1970* The Stationery Office ISBN 0 10 544170 8

43 *The Sex Discrimination Act 1975* The Stationery Office ISBN 0 10 546575 5

HSE priced and free publications are available by mail order from HSE Books, PO Box 1999, Sudbury, Suffolk CO10 2WA
Tel: 01787 881165
Fax: 01787 313995
Website: www.hsebooks.co.uk
(HSE priced publications are also available from bookshops.)

The Stationery Office (formerly HMSO) publications are available from The Publications Centre, PO Box 276, London SW8 5DT
Tel: 0870 600 5522
Fax: 0870 600 5533
Website: www.tso.co.uk
(They are also available from bookshops.)

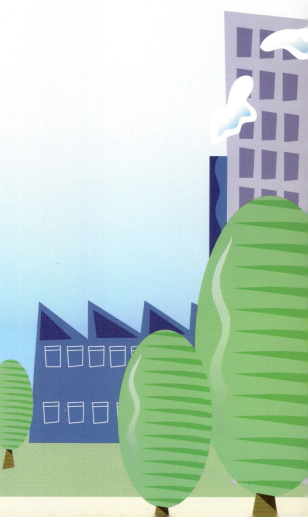

# Sources of help

HSE Information Services
Caerphilly Business Park
Caerphilly
CF83 3GG
Tel: 08701 545500
Fax: 02920 859260
email:
hseinformationservices@natbrit.com
Website: www.hse.gov.uk

Department for Work and Pensions
Public Enquiry Office
The Adelphi
1-11 John Adam Street
London
WC2N 6HT
Tel: 020 7712 2171
Fax: 020 7712 2386
Website: www.dwp.gov.uk

Department of Trade and Industry
Enquiry Unit
1 Victoria Street
London
SW1H 0ET
Tel: 020 7215 5000
email: enquiries@dti.gsi.gov.uk
Websites: www.dti.gov.uk;
www.tiger.gov.uk

Department for Transport
Enquiry Service
Great Minster House
76 Marsham Street
London
SW1P 4DR
Tel: 020 7944 8300
Fax: 020 7944 6589
Website: www.dft.gov.uk

Equal Opportunities Commission
Arndale House, Arndale Centre
Manchester
M4 3EQ
Tel: 0845 601 5901
Fax: 0161 838 1733
email: info@eoc.org.uk
Website: www.eoc.org.uk

The Maternity Alliance
45 Beech Street
London
EC2P 2LX
Tel: 020 7588 8582
Fax: 020 7588 8584
Website: www.maternityalliance.org.uk

Tommys the Baby Charity
1 Kennington Road
London
SE1 7RR
Tel: 08707 707070
Fax: 020 7928 6628
e-mail: mailbox@tommys.org
Website: www.tommys.org

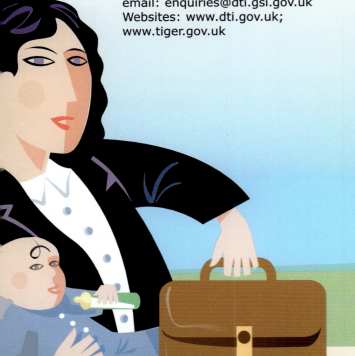

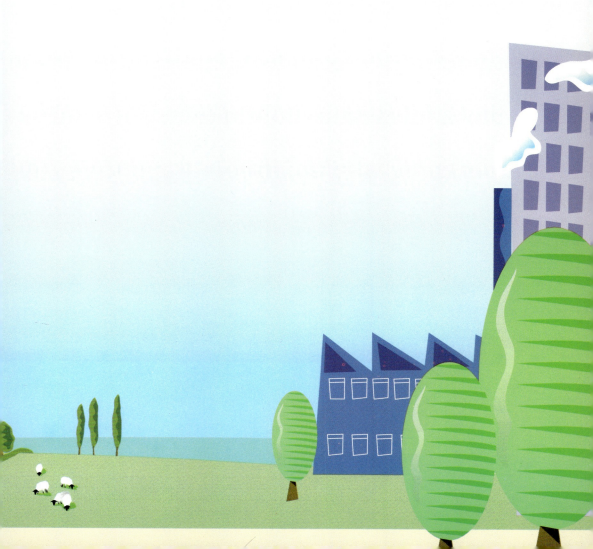

**New and expectant mothers at work**
A guide for employers

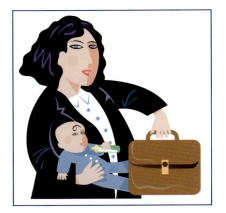

Printed and published by the Health and Safety Executive

**C100    11/02**